Intermittent Fasting

For Health and Fast Fat Loss

By Shawn Reath

Introduction

I want to thank you and congratulate you for downloading the book, *"Intermittent Fasting for Health and Fast Fat Loss."*

This book contains proven steps and strategies on how to become healthy and lose fat faster through intermittent fasting. It is going to show you the benefits of intermittent fasting and explain why it is better than diets, liposuction or any fat loss method. Then it is going to show you several ways of doing intermittent fasting and how easy these are.

Other diets have a strict regimen of foods to eat frequently or to avoid altogether. Some diets require certain food combinations. Others ask that you put in several hours of activity. Almost all will impose some restrictions that leave you light-headed, dizzy or always hungry. Unfortunately not all diets provide the results they guarantee. That's why you end up quitting with very little to show for all the trouble and effort.

Intermittent fasting will not disappoint you. It is scientific with proven claims. It is all natural and takes into account what you can and are willing to do. It will not have any severe impositions nor will it have any adverse side effects. The only thing you will see with intermittent fasting is the improvement of your health and fast fat loss.

Thanks again for downloading this book, I hope you enjoy it!

Why You Should Read This Book

This book will help you finally find the best solution to health and fast fat loss. If you have been disappointed by the claims of other diets, then that is one good reason to read this book. This book is going to tell you what is missing from all those diets and why should consider intermittent fasting instead.

Another reason to read this book is if you are exhausted by the restrictions and impositions made by other diets. You will be surprised that intermittent fasting doesn't tell you what food to avoid or eat frequently. Yet you will discover that you are able to lose fat fast and become healthier. Does that mean you can gorge on cholesterol-laden, high fat and high carb junk food? Read and find out.

Finally, if you are still searching for a reason to read this book, read it for the pleasure of discovering that being healthy and losing fat fast is not something complicated, restrictive or bland-tasting. Read this book to understand what intermittent fasting really is. You will be delighted to discover that it is a fun way to enjoy your favorite food and still lose weight and become a fitter person.

Copyright

Disclaimer

The information provided in this book is designed to provide helpful information
on the subjects discussed. This book is not meant to be used, nor should it be used, to
diagnose or treat any medical condition. For diagnosis or treatment of any medical
problem, consult your own physician. The publisher and author are not responsible for
any specific health or allergy needs that may require medical supervision and are not
liable for any damages or negative consequences from any treatment, action, application
or preparation, to any person reading or following the information in this book. Any
references included are provided for informational purposes only and do not constitute
endorsement of any websites or other sources. Readers should be aware that any websites
listed in this book may change.

Table of Contents

Intermittent Fasting – What is it?

Fasting is basically going without food or nourishment for a period of time. Did you know that most, if not all, people fast without being compelled to? They do that every night when they go to sleep. Sleeping for 6 to eat hours is basically fasting.

Fasting is not something new. For millennia, people of all faiths and beliefs use it as part of their worship and religious ritual. For instance, Christ said to have fasted for 40 days, Buddha ate only one seed a day while meditating for enlightenment, Muslims fast daily for a month during Ramadan, while the Mormons fast every first Sunday of the month. The goals of such ritual are to discipline the body and control all worldly appetites, passions and desires.

Outside of sleep and the religious significance, pre-historic men practiced fasting regularly since they did not have easy access to food back then. As foragers and hunters, Paleolithic men ate only when they found fruit or caught game. In fact, the concept of breakfast or eating three square meals did not happen until they discovered how to grow and raise their own food. Even then, most ancient farmers ate only once or twice a day with as long as 8 to 12 hours in between. Then, as ideas and concepts on food and nutrition evolved, the custom of eating several meals all day in order to keep from feeling hungry became prevalent. Science supported this notion by suggesting that eating many small meals is a good way to maintain high metabolic rates. Further research also suggested having a big breakfast in order have all the nutrients and energy needed to sustain a day's work. Even today, that thought process still guides proponents of Paleo and other diets even though current research questions the validity and logic of having big breakfast and multiple meals.

In 1939, scientists began studying fasting and its benefits. They started to look at cultures that only had one mid-day meal; they also studied other forms of non-religious fasting like skipping breakfast or eating sparingly on certain days. The results of their studies indicate that increasing the duration between meals actually has more benefits to health and fat loss than eating only certain food. They discovered that when people ate as much as they wanted for five days and then eat little for the remaining two, they actually experienced faster fat loss without risk to health. These findings helped introduced the concept of intermittent fasting.

So what is intermittent fasting?

Intermittent fasting is a term used to describe fasting by schedules. Simply put it is eating normally for a certain period followed by periods of eating sparingly or not at all. As the term "intermittent" implies, this fasting is periodic rather than random otherwise it throws your metabolism into disarray. Proponents such as Dr. Mosley, author of *The Fast Diet: Lose Weight, Stay Healthy, and Live Longer with the Simple Secret of Intermittent Fasting,* suggest that intermittent fasting involves cutting your calorie intake a couple of days a week. Other advocates suggest similar schedules such as making that every other day or having just a single nightly meal.

Intermittent fasting doesn't tell you what to eat or avoid, making it more like a lifestyle change rather than a diet. It also asks you to change your eating habits by altering your mealtime schedules and reducing the amount of food you eat. This makes it easier to follow without the aggravated symptoms of a diet change such as flatulence, light-headedness, cravings or hunger pangs. This is most interesting since most people expect fasting to encourage binge eating. Studies however show that while that does happen occasionally, most folks who practice intermittent fasting do not seem to suffer any ill effects at all. In fact, their energy levels on days they fast are almost the same as when they aren't.

Dieting advocates the reduction of carb, fat and proteins. Intermittent fasting only recommends a reduction of total calorie intake. It does not impose a list of forbidden food although some IF practitioners call for eating healthier food rather than gorging on junk.

The key to the success of intermittent fasting is forcing the body to go through a cycle of fullness and want. This cycle is what forces the body's metabolism to feed off fat reserves rather than sugar for energy; and this causes fat loss and makes intermittent fasting ideal for anyone who wants to lose weight without dietary restrictions. In fact, some athletes and body builders go through a regimen of intermittent fasting to get rid of fat before normalizing their diet or embarking on a weight-training program.

Intermittent fasting leaves out the religious or spiritual rituals. It does not require yoga exercises, deep pondering, meditation or anything similar to curb hunger. Most advocates however advocate seeing a doctor before embarking on any type of intermittent fasting in order to avoid unnecessary risks. Pregnant or nursing women as well as people with certain health conditions such as diabetes, hypoglycemia or any disorder that requires you not to go below a certain calorie range, should not consider intermittent fasting. Obese people with heart conditions might also need to reconsider intermittent fasting as a means to better health and fast fat loss.

So is intermittent fasting for you?

Benefits of Intermittent Fasting

In order to better understand if intermittent fasting is the solution you are looking for to stay healthy and lost fat fast, examine the following benefits:

Restoration of Fat as the Body's Fuel

Your body currently uses sugar as its primary source of fuel as the result of eating gluten-rich grain products and sugar-rich processed food. Sugar as a fuel is inefficient and produces undesirable products such as free radicals. Research shows that intermittent fasting restores fat as the body's primary fuel. This is because fasting forces your body to utilize its fat deposits when its sugar sources are low due to decrease or absence of food. Fasting also induces the secretion of such hormones as HGH. HGH or the human growth hormone, burns off fat cells in order to provide your body energy.

Through intermittent fasting, your body learns to recognize periods where sugar sources are low so it programs metabolizing your fat reserves instead of sugar. As long as you do not binge on sugar foods after your fast or make your fasting days random and infrequent, your body will continue using fat. When that happens the natural consequence is for your body to fast fat lose making you trimmer and leaner quickly.

Reduction of Sugar Dependence

As you continue to fast intermittently, your body becomes accustomed to burning fat rather than sugar as fuel. This makes you naturally less dependent on sugar. That in turn suppresses your cravings for sweets and the appetite for snacks. You rely less on a sugar "high" to give you an energy boost and you become less prone to chronic diseases such as diabetes, hypertension, stroke etc.

Normalization of Insulin Sensitivity

When your body regularly consumes sugar in levels found in processed and junk food, your body is forced to use it as fuel. It also induces a biochemical reaction in your body called insulin resistance. Insulin resistance causes the cells of the body to leak glucose, fat and amino acids. This decreases energy production, which is why you feel weak and drained after a "sugar rush." Far worse, insulin resistance increases the risk of chronic disease such as heart disease or even cancer.

Fasting drops your sugar sources and normalizes the sensitivity of your body's cells to insulin. This improves the cell's mitochondrial energy production and reduces leptin resistance. Leptin is a hormone tied closely to insulin levels and functions to regulate fat metabolism. Insulin resistance induces leptin resistance which makes your body increase fat cells rather than burn them for energy. By fasting intermittently, you force leptin to be secreted, curb insulin and leptin resistance and use your body's fat reserves.

Normalization of the Hunger Hormone

The hunger hormone known as ghrelin is controls your cravings and desire to eat. Ghrelin serves to balance your body's energy stores as well as your weight. For instance, if you lose weight your ghrelin level rises causing you to eat more to gain it back. On the other hand, as soon as you gain weight, your ghrelin levels drops and you lose appetite and the desire to eat more. Sugar consumption inhibits normal ghrelin function and causes you to continue eating. However, intermittent fasting restores ghrelin's normal function and allows your ghrelin levels to rise and fall regularly. This makes eating and fasting normal and in turn, causes fast fat loss through metabolism.

Deceleration of Aging

As mentioned above, intermittent fasting provokes the secretion of the human growth hormone. This hormone not only burns fat, it also promotes muscle growth and repair, bone build-up and skin tightening. These processes slow down aging and make people look and feel younger. Indeed, research show that men who fast intermittently produce human growth hormones by as much as 2000 percent while women produce 1,400 percent. This boost in HGH production prevents the skin from sagging once the fat stores are gone. It also results into greater endurance with faster recovery from muscle fatigue. This allows you to exercise more and build a younger looking physique.

Fasting also decreases the production of free radicals and their accumulation in the body's cells. It does these by suppressing oxidative stress due to aging and preventing lipids, nucleic acids and cell proteins from being damaged by the aging process. The result is improved skin tone and lighter and flexible movements.

Finally, the normalization of insulin sensitivity along with the inhibition of the mTOR pathway through fasting slows down aging and contributes to a more youthful look.

Prevention of Disease

Fasting's normalization of ghrelin, insulin and leptin creates a domino effect through the body that decreases excessive and chronic inflammation as well as oxidative stress. This in turn suppresses the proliferation of free radicals and the cellular damage they cause which often leads to chronic disease and cancer. Fasting also lowers the levels of triglycerides through the metabolism of fat cells, which is a disease biomarker. This means that the lower your levels of triglycerides are, the less you expose yourself to the risk of diabetes, hypertension and obesity. Fasting also regulates blood sugar levels through improved insulin sensitivity. Blood sugar is a biomarker that indicates your risk to debilitating diseases like diabetes depending on how high or low its level is.

Research has shown that decreasing food consumption through fasting reduces the risk of many diseases by as much as 30 percent. In fact data has shown that fasting not only reduced the incidence of disease in animals but it also caused an increase in longevity.

Prevention of Psychological Deterioration

Research and scientific studies on the benefits of intermittent fasting suggest its use in the possible treatment and prevention of dementia, Parkinson's and even depression. This due to two substances produced through fasting: ketones and BDNF.

Ketone is the brain's preferred fuel instead of glucose. The production of ketones goes into overdrive when fasting forces the body to burn fat. Ketones enable the production of mitochondria and increase glutathione levels in the region of the brain called the hippocampus. Natural glutathione is a very powerful antioxidant that protects the brain from inflammation and infection. This makes it crucial in the treatment and potential prevention of depression. Ketones also stimulate the growth of new neural pathways in the brain that helps Alzheimer patients.

BDNF or brain-derived neurotropic factor is a protein produced through intermittent fasting. BDNF converts the stem cells of the brain into new neurons. It also triggers several biochemical reactions that improve neural health and protects the brain from cellular changes caused by Parkinson's, Huntington's and Alzheimer's. Research conducted by the National Institute on Aging confirm that as much as 50 to 400 percent increase in BDNF can be expected by simply fasting or cutting down calorie intake to as low as 600 calories every other day.

Detoxification

One of the effects of a poor diet is it hinders the autophagy process. This is the body's natural way of cleansing and replacing worn out parts of the cell particularly in the mitochondria. Even a healthy diet can interfere with autophagy by putting it in a constant state of digestion. Through intermittent fasting, the body is able to execute the autophagy process and apply cleansing and detoxification at the cellular level.

Intermittent fasting also increases autophagy and eliminating worn out mitochondria as well as other damaged cellular particles from the neurons. This makes intermittent fasting a potential therapeutic treatment for such neuron centric ailments as Parkinson's, Huntington's, dementia and Alzheimer's.

The 5:2 Intermittent Fasting

With the various benefits of intermittent fasting, how should one begin?

There are many methods and techniques for intermittent fasting. Among the more popular as well as earlier techniques is one recommended by Dr. Mosley, author of the book, *The Fast Diet: Lose Weight, Stay Healthy, and Live Longer with the Simple Secret of Intermittent Fasting*. The method Dr. Mosley recommends in his book is as the 5:2 intermittent fasting plan.

The 5:2 intermittent fasting is simple. All you need to do is divide the week into five days for eating normally and 2 days for fasting. You can have two days of eating normally followed by a day of fasting then two more days of normal eating. Your sixth day will be your day of fasting followed by a day of normal eating. Another version of this fast is to eat as low as 400-500 calories a day for the first day then eat as much as 2000-2500 calories for the next 2 days. You then repeat the same cycle for the remaining days of the week.

On normal days, Dr Mosley makes no recommendations for any food variety to skip or eat in lesser quantities. He doesn't make the same recommendation on fasting days. However, he suggests reducing your meals to 500-600 calories or about a fourth of what you eat normally. He also suggests accompanying that with lots of zero-calorie tea or water to stave off hunger pangs.

Eating only 400 to 500 calories may be tough. To make it easier for people to get through their fast days, some advocates of intermittent fasting suggest having smoothies or shakes. You might want to have a smoothie that packed with antioxidants and nutrients with less carbs and proteins. This will enable you to sip and slurp rather than have a very small meal. Then when your body has adjusted to the schedule of fasting, you can swap your smoothie for a more solid snack such as a handful of nuts, a fruit cup, banana or a serving of fish or meat.

The 5:2 intermittent fasting schedule is great if you want to lose weight. The huge cuts in your food intake can net you a weight loss of two to two and a half pounds a week. In fact, Dr. Mosley claims he lost a total of 19 pounds in 2 months by just following the 5:2 intermittent fast method.

Among the things to watch out for using this method is the possibility of binge eating especially during days when you eat normally. Avoid this by planning your meals ahead of time. You can even plan which restaurants you go to or where to eat during normal and fast days. It is also important that you align your work schedule so that way your fast doesn't fall on a day when you get invited to an all you can eat dinner buffet.

Eat-Stop-Eat Intermittent Fasting

Another form of intermittent fasting made popular by Brad Pilon, a leading expert and author if *Eat Stop Eat,* is suggested by the book title is, "Eat Stop Eat."

This form of fasting is simple. All you need to do is fast completely for 24 hours at least one or two days a week. During this fast, you do not eat at all, not even snacks. You may however have water or any calorie free beverage. As soon as the fast is over, you start eating normally until the next fast.

Most of those who begin this form of intermittent fasting complain that 24 hours without food is a long time. However, Pilon explains that this program is flexible and people can choose to start their fast by going as long as they are able before breaking it. They can do this by including sleep time as part of the fast. They can also start with half a day and gradually increase the length of time they fast until they are able to do a full day. He also suggests scheduling the fast on a day without any eating obligations such as business dinners, work lunches, happy hours, or any kind of occasion. Finally, he suggests acting as if you're not fasting to prevent any cravings or hunger pangs from making you break it.

Practitioners of this method of intermittent fasting suggest beginning the fast after dinner while others suggest having it after lunch so that you only skip two meals instead of three.

Whatever, the method, the important thing per Pilon, is not to snack or eat anything during the 24-hour fasting period. The only thing that you can take is a glass of water or anything without calories. Doing this will really drive your metabolism to burn fat and detoxify.

One good thing with this method is it removes the need to count calories or measure portions during the fast while avoiding certain foods during the non-fast periods. However, Pilon cautions against over-eating or going on a free-for-all after fasting. People who try the eat-stop-eat should eat like adults and consume food that is nutritionally balanced and healthy especially if the goal is a good health and not just fast fat loss. The temptation of binge eating after a fast is one of two drawbacks of this method. The other drawback is because of the longer fasting period, most people struggle with going through extended periods of having no food. This causes them to suffer fatigue, headaches, anxiety or irritability and crankiness. Some people are able to overcome these symptoms as they continue to practice these but most fail.

Other Intermittent Fasting Options

In addition to the two fasting methods, here are a few variations you might want to consider.

Leangain

If you go to the gym often and want to lose that fat fast and build muscle, you might want to consider the Leangain intermittent fasting developed by Martain Beckhan.

This method divides the day into "fasting" and "feeding" period. The "fasting" period is typically 14 hours for women and 16 hours for men during where there is no calorie consumption whatsoever. You may however consume diet soda, calorie-free drinks, black coffee or chew sugarless gum. Almost everyone who follows this method recommends beginning the fast at night and has their first meal usually four to 6 hours after waking up.

"Feeding" time is about usually between the remaining eight to ten hours of the day and can be broken into three meals. Leangains allows the fasting schedule to be adaptable anyone but requires that the feeding window remain consistent. This is important in order to make following the program easier and avoid hormonal imbalance. It is also important to watch what you eat and match it with the type of workout you are doing. This means making sure you have carb-rich food during the days you exercise. You should eat more fat during rest days and make sure you get protein every day. You should base your protein intake on the workout goals and activity levels as well as your age, gender and body fat. Leangains is the only intermittent fasting method that requires you to make sure you eat whole, unprocessed foods. It does allow you to have why-based protein shakes or a protein bar if you have no time for a nutritious meal.

If you choose to follow leangains, you have the flexibility to eat anytime within your feeding window. However, you have to adhere to specific guidelines on meals and nutrition in relation to your workout schedule.

Warrior's Diet

A variation to the leangain method of intermittent fasting is the Warriors Diet. This diet slash fasting schedule has a longer fasting period as much as 20 hours a day. Feeding period is for the remaining hours at night and should consist of only one large meal, this came from the philosophy that humans eat best at night. Thus, the idea of a eating a large meal of specific food is to ensure that your body gets the nutrients it needs in harmony with your circadian cycle. It is therefore very important to watch what you eat to make sure it is protein-packed, carb-rich and nutrient-heavy. This takes advantage of the ability of Parasympathetic Nervous System to promote calm, digestion and relaxation while helping the body recover and recuperate.

During the fasting period of The Warrior Diet, you can eat small servings of fresh raw vegetables or fruit. You may also drink some fresh juice or eat a small serving of meat or fish for protein in order to stimulate the "flight or fight" response of the Sympathetic Nervous System and boost alertness, energy and the burning of fat.

Many weight watchers and athletes prefer this method to others because it reportedly speeds up fat loss and increases energy. It also allows some eating during the "fasting" period. However, the strict guidelines on what and when to eat make this difficult to follow for life. Only those dedicated enough to give up activities that interfere with the fasting and feeding schedules and enjoy following strict guidelines on eating, appreciate the Warriors Diet. It is certainly not for anyone who does not prefer eating large meals at night.

Alternate Day Fasting

Finally, for anyone looking to try out an easy intermittent fasting method, the alternate day fasting is the perfect choice. Just like the 5:2, alternate day fasting means eating as lows one fifth of your normal meals one day, and eat normally the next. This method allows eating smoothies or sipping meal replacement shakes instead of having smaller meals during "fast" days. However, this is only good for the first two weeks and efforts should be done to transition to a meal of solid food. This will ensure that your metabolism stays on track and keeps burning fat as fuel instead of glycogen from your muscle cells.

This is by and large one of the easier intermittent fasting methods for everyone to follow in order to achieve good health and fast fat loss.

Additional Tips for Intermittent Fasting

Has the previous chapter challenged you to give intermittent fasting a try?

If so here are a few tips to keep in mind:

Hydrate

Drinking plenty of water during your fasting period, regardless if it is for 14 hours or an entire day, makes it easier to get through the absence of food. Avoid drinking coffee and diuretics that make you lose water and crave for something solid.

Begin fasting at night

This makes fasting easier because it takes advantage of sleep to mitigate eight hours of missing food. Fasting through the night also takes advantage of your circadian rhythm to enable metabolism and allow cellular detoxification to take place.

Fast when you are busy

It is easier to fast when your mind is preoccupied with something other than food or when you are too busy to think of having a snack. This is why you should plan to begin fasting when you are busy rather than when you are lounging in front of the TV. Chances are the lack of activity and food is just going to increase your craving for a snack. That said, you should engage in something that requires energy, but is low intensity. This is not saying you should get on a workout when you're fasting. However, some low intensity cardio exercises will do you no harm.

Think of Fasting as a break

Brad Pilon, creator of the Eat-Stop-Eat intermittent fasting method suggests thinking about fasting as a break rather than a deprivation. This changes your perspective and allows your mind to stop worrying about what and when to eat next. This also establishes the correct mindset to pursue long-term intermittent fasting plans and allow you to follow guidelines and plan meals. Also, by picturing fasting as a break, you are setting up your body to follow a pattern rather than react to starvation.

Exercise

When you accompany regular exercise with intermittent fasting you get better results. You do not need to engage in serious hardcore workouts or weight training. You can do muscle toning or full-body strength training during your normal or "feeding" periods at least twice or thrice a week.

Here are a few tips to remember when you exercise in order maximize fast fat loss:

Do low-intensity cardio when you are fasting
You can perform cardio exercises when you are fasting. Just make sure they are low-intensity, meaning you are able to carry out a conversation and not gasp for breath while exercising in the middle of your fast. A slightly brisk walk or a light jog are sufficient exercises and should not get you into trouble. However, pay close attention to your body and stop exercising if you start to run short of breath, feel dizzy, light-headed or nauseous. You should not exercise too hard or too long or it could do you more harm than good. The low intensity cardio will get your metabolism going and hasten fat loss.

Do high-intensity workouts after you have eaten.
In order to maximize losing fat while having lots of energy, intermittent fasting programs recommend that you schedule your workouts as close to your last meal. Leangains for instance, has strict guidelines that any workout sessions of moderate to high intensity should take place around your last meal. This is to ensure you have sufficient glycogen to burn as you workout. This will also reduce the risk of making your blood sugar level too low.

Always have a snack rich in carbs to replenish your body's depleted fuel sources after you complete any high-intensity workout. This will continue to ensure your body doesn't switch from burning fat to burning glycogen.

Load up on protein.
Regular consumption of protein-rich food is critical before and after weight training especially if you are looking at building muscle mass. Having a pre-workout snack helps give your body fuel but you need protein for muscle synthesis throughout the day. It is especially critical to load up on protein right after your workout in order for your muscles to grow and repair themselves. According to the Academy of Nutrition and Dietetics, your body needs to ingest 20 to 30 grams of high-quality protein every four of your waking hours and after working out in order to maximize muscle growth.

It is important when doing intermittent fasting that you schedule any strength training workouts between two meals, a meal and a snack, or at least between two snacks. Always make sure that your food provides you with sufficient protein.

The importance of loading up on protein ensures that the body continues burning fat as its primary source of fuel and prevents it from cannibalizing on muscles for glycogen.

Take advantage of snacks.
Take advantage of the flexibility that intermittent fasting allows about eating snacks and meals. Consuming a snack or a meal 3 -4 hours before

you hit the gym ensures that you will have enough energy to complete your workout. If you are prone to run low on blood sugar, make sure to snack one to two hours before exercising. Make sure your snack or meal has proteins that will stable your blood sugar level and some fast-acting carbs. Make sure that you eat something with at least 20 grams of carbs and 20 grams of protein within two hours of completing your workout to replenish your glycogen stores, build-up your muscles and keep you energized.

Having a snack will ensure that sugars are not reintroduced and that your body's metabolism keeps burning fat.

As you follow these tips, whatever intermittent fasting method you follow whether that's Warrior diet or alternating days, will cause your body to burn fat for your energy needs. This will shrink the size of your body's fat cells. It will reduce cellulite build-up in your butt and thighs and it will continue to improve your physique and health. Fast fat loss now becomes a reality within days of trying out intermittent fasting. This loss will become eminent when you measure the number of pounds you shed in just a few weeks.

Bonus Chapter - Precautions

Intermittent fasting while appropriate for most, may pose some risks especially to people with hypoglycemia or diabetes. Hypoglycemia is a condition where your blood sugar drops to an abnormally low level. It is often associated with diabetes but that is not often the case. Some people have hypoglycemia even if they do not have a history of diabetes or previously diagnosed with it. It is therefore very critical that you check with your doctor before embarking on a fast or even a reduced eating program.

If you are fasting and you begin experiencing such symptoms as headaches, tremors, irritation, sudden hunger and weakness, you just might be having a hypoglycemic crash. You will know your blood sugar levels are dropping to a severe low if your symptoms start to include the following: seizures, double or blurred vision, increasing confusion, any abnormal behavior, and finally, loss of consciousness.

Ideally, you should not get into intermittent fasting if you have hypoglycemia. Instead, you should work on normalizing your blood sugar. You can do this by eliminating sugars and grains from your diet. Replace these with foods packed with healthy fat and high quality proteins. For instance, swap bread for coconut oil and healthy fats. Coconut oil is a good substitute for sugar because it does not require insulin and can be rapidly metabolized making it ideal to use once you start fasting. In fact, if you suspect that you are on the verge of a hypoglycemic crash, take some coconut oil as a preventive measure. However, understand that it will take some time before your blood sugar normalizes so don't plunge right back into exercise or fasting.

People with adrenal fatigue or chronic stress as well as pregnant or nursing women would also need to avoid fasting and instead, focus on improving nutrition through a diet of organic food packed with healthy fat and high-quality protein.

Bonus Chapter from the Book "5:2 Diet"

Benefits of 5:2 Intermittent Fasting

So is the 5:2 Diet or method of intermittent fasting for you? In order to better understand if it is, examine the following benefits:

5:2 offers a manageable schedule of fasting

Intermittent fasting employs fasting by schedules. From the comparisons done on the other methods, 5:2 would have the simplest and most manageable schedule. A person shifting from a normal non-fasting daily schedule will not be stymied by a 14-36 fasting hour period that can be stressful. On the other hand, the two full days of fasting that comes with 6:2 will not be too difficult to follow especially since the person is still allowed a small meal. This means that metabolism, insulin, leptin, and ghrelin levels will not go awry or experience a drastic change. The extremes of a single large meal or a daily longer period for fasting which usually breaks the back of anyone who wants to try out intermittent fasting will not be encountered.

Manageable Weight Loss

The 5:2 intermittent fasting method is a wonderful way to lose weight. The drop in 23 days out of 5 is sufficient to stimulate fat burning that will have the net effect losing two to two and a half pounds a week. In fact Dr. Michael Mosley, proponent of the 5:2 diet has revealed that he has lost 19 pounds in just 2 months of following the 5:2 intermittent fasting method. This is because intermittent fasting forces the body to go through a metabolic cycle that feeds off its fat reserves. Fasting triggers ketosis which in turn causes fat burning. Additional hormonal releases such as HGH trigger further fat utilization.

Dr. Mosley's experience confirms the findings of studies as early as 1939 when scientists started researching the benefits of fasting. Their findings from cultural observations on non-religious fasting indicated that a longer duration between meals actually produce better health and weight loss than dieting, They specifically discovered that individuals who fasted twice a week then ate whatever they wanted for the remaining period had lesser risks to health and faster fat loss.

Lifestyle Change

Unlike diets which are essentially meal plans and lists of what to eat or avoid, intermittent fasting is a lifestyle change that requires you to modify eating schedules and skipping or reducing the amount of food eaten. This requires if necessary a change in schedule to ensure that activities are not affected by the switch to fasting such as weekend dinners, bar hopping, or dining out. It also necessitates an additional change in activities such as exercise, physical activities and working from home.

The lifestyle changes allow you to cope up with the initial symptoms of fasting until it becomes easy to follow. The 5:2 intermittent fasting method makes it even easier to do as it has less of the symptoms of diet change like cravings, flatulence, irritability, light-headedness or hunger pangs. It also does not automatically lead to binge eating. In fact, most adherents of 5:2 rarely fall into binge eating and their energy levels remain constant whether they fast or not.

Better Health

Even though intermittent fasting recommends a reduction of total calories consumed rather than a ban on certain food, it still results into better health. This is because of the following:

Disease Prevention

Because intermittent fasting normalizes insulin, ghrelin, and leptin levels, it causes the body to decrease oxidative stress and chronic excessive inflammation which in turn cause free radical accumulation and cell and tissue damage. This suppresses the risk of debilitating diseases like hypertension, diabetes and even cancer.

5:2 intermittent fasting can regularly lower triglycerides levels by metabolizing fat cells which lowers the risk of contracting stroke, hypertension, obesity and diabetes. It also improves insulin sensitivity which improves your blood sugar levels and with it your risk of avoiding diabetes or cardiovascular diseases.

Statistical analysis of the effects of intermittent fasting indicates that it decreases the risk of food-related diseases by as much as 30 percent with a corresponding increase in longevity.

Improves Mental Health

Scientific studies on intermittent fasting identified that the production of ketones when the body starts metabolizing fat enables new growth of mitochondria and an increase of glutathione in the hippocampus of the brain protecting it from infection and inflammation. This makes fasting a potential tool in the treatment of dementia, depression and even Parkinson's. Ketones can also grow new neural pathways making fasting another potential tool for the treatment of Alzheimer's.

Fasting also produces brain-derived neurotropic factor or BDNF which converts the brain's stem cells into new neurons which protect the brain from cellular changes due to Alzheimer's, Huntington's and Parkinson's diseases. According to the National Institute on Aging simple fasting or reduces one's consumption to 600 calories every other day can increase BDNF levels by as much as 400 percent.

Anti-aging

When intermittent fasting stimulates the secretion of HGH or the human growth hormone, it metabolizes fat, promotes muscle repair and growth and tightens the skin. This anti-aging effect makes people feel and look younger than they really are. Indeed, research has shown that fasting intermittently, boosts HGH production in women by 1400 percent and in men by 2000. This results into faster recovery from muscle fatigue, greater physical endurance and automatic skin tightening which produces a slender, younger looking physique.

The 5:2 intermittent fasting method can decrease free radical production by preventing further damage to cell proteins, nucleic acids and lipids due to oxidative stress and the aging process. Finally, it also normalizes insulin sensitivity and inhibits the mTOR pathway to slow down aging, resulting in a more youthful glow.

5:2 Intermittent Fasting FAQ's

Before you try out the 5:2 Diet or intermittent fasting method, here are a few FAQ's to keep in mind:

Can you begin fasting after dinner?

Fasting can be done by anyone and there is nothing wrong to start your fast after dinner. This will just make fasting easier because it takes advantage of sleep and your circadian rhythm to metabolize and allow cellular detoxification to take place.

When should I fast?

Fast at a time when your mind is busy and you are too preoccupied to think about eating. This means don't begin fasting when you are relaxing on a weekend. Chances are the lack of food and activity will force you to want to eat more than you are allowed to.

That said, don't schedule fast days on a weekend, holiday, or for that matter on Friday dinners, Monday brunches, or social events. You should either have a good excuse to miss these activities or revise your schedule.

Can I Exercise?

You certainly can perform regular exercise during your fast days. Evidence suggests that there is no risk to health when you do. Just do not engage in serious weight training or hard core work outs. Here are a couple of guidelines to remember in order to make exercise work:

> **Perform low-intensity cardio when fasting**
> When fasting, limit exercises to low-intensity cardio routines such as a brisk walk or a light jog. These are sufficient exercises and should not get you into trouble. You can do upper body exercises, squats, splits, pushups but make sure you are able to carry out a conversation in mid-exercising. Pay close attention to how you feel and stop exercising if you start to run short of breath, feel light-headed or dizzy. Don't increase the intensity or it could do you more harm than good. Low intensity cardio should be sufficient to jumpstart your metabolism.
>
> Drink water to keep hydrated during your work out.
>
> **Do high-intensity workouts after you have eaten.**
> Maximize fat loss while having lots of energy by scheduling your workouts as close to your last meal. Feel free to have workout sessions of moderate to high intensity including weight training. This will ensure you have sufficient glycogen to burn as you workout.

Have a carb-rich snack to replenish your body's depleted fuel sources after you complete any high-intensity workout to avoid switching from burning fat to burning glycogen. Make sure you eat protein-rich food before and after your workouts as well and that you are well-nourished before starting another fasting session. Never do intermittent fasting unless your workouts are well within your feast days. Sandwich them between two snacks, a snack and a meal or two meals and always make sure to load up on carbs and protein.

Can I have a snack while fasting?

Take advantage of the flexibility that intermittent fasting allows with regard to eating snacks and meals. Consuming a snack or a meal 3 -4 hours before you hit the gym ensures that you will have enough energy to complete your workout. If you are prone to run low on blood sugar, make sure to snack one to two hours before exercising. Make sure your snack or meal has proteins that will stable your blood sugar level and some fast-acting carbs. Make sure that you eat something with at least 20 grams of carbs and 20 grams of protein within two hours of completing your workout to replenish your glycogen stores, build-up your muscles and keep you energized.

Having such a snack will ensure that sugars are not reintroduced and that your body's metabolism keeps burning fat.

As you follow these tips, whatever intermittent fasting method you follow whether that's Warrior diet or alternating days, will cause your body to burn fat for your energy needs. This will shrink the size of your body's fat cells. It will reduce cellulite build-up in your butt and thighs and it will continue to improve your physique and health. Fast fat loss now becomes a reality within days of trying out intermittent fasting. This loss will become eminent when you measure the number of pounds you shed in just a few weeks.

Who should avoid the 5:2 Diet?

While the 5:2 intermittent fasting us relatively low risk, it is still important to see a doctor before attempting to fast if only to avoid unwanted risks. Women who are pregnant as well as those nursing a child should not consider fasting. The same is true with people afflicted by diabetes or hypoglycemia. In fact any illness that requires you avoid eating below a certain range of calories should make you think twice about fasting. Obese people suffering from heart problems and other organ issues should seek further advice from a doctor before considering intermittent fasting as a means of achieving weight loss and better health. People with adrenal fatigue or chronic stress should also avoid intermittent fasting.

Conclusion

So have you decided on intermittent fasting and picked out which method to use?

Are you convinced that it promotes better health and fast fat loss compared to other diets?

Except for a few people such as those with hypoglycemia, chronic stress, or are currently pregnant or nursing a baby, intermittent fasting is applicable to anyone. If you want to use it to cut down fat and bulk up, you have the Warrior's diet or leangains. If you think that one meal a day and long daily fasts are unbearable you have Eat-Stop-Eat or 5:2. And if that is still too difficult for you, you have alternate-day intermittent fasting.

All of these programs are flexible enough to accommodate your needs especially if exercise and food restrictions are not your type.

The next step is to review the different intermittent fasting methods and see which one aligns best with your goal of health and fast fat loss. Check with your doctor if there are any risks to your health such as hypoglycemia or chronic stress. Then if necessary, make the appropriate correction needed to normalize.

Once you are in a position to start intermittent fasting, there are no other restrictions or impositions. Just be consistent with the times that you eat. If you are doing a workout, remember the tips on exercise to maximize fat loss without losing energy. Remember to snack or eat something with protein before work outs and don't forget to do the same afterwards.

You will be surprised at how quickly you lose fat and gain good health.

One Last Thing...

If you enjoyed this book or found it useful I'd be very grateful if you'd post a short review on Amazon. Your support really does make a difference and I read all the reviews personally so I can get your feedback and make this book even better.

If you'd like to leave a review then all you need to do is click the review link on this book's page...

Thank You so Much